Book Description

With this book, you will walk away with a basic understanding of the ketogenic diet, associated vocabulary, and how it affects the body overall.

Keto Diet Basics

Beginner's Guide to Burning Fat, Losing Weight, Lowering Inflammation, and Improving Anxiety & Depression by Learning What the Ketogenic Diet Really Is… (And Isn't)

Jordan Casey

© Copyright 2021 - All rights reserved.

The content contained within this book may not be reproduced, duplicated or transmitted without direct written permission from the author or the publisher.

Under no circumstances will any blame or legal responsibility be held against the publisher, or author, for any damages, reparation, or monetary loss due to the information contained within this book, either directly or indirectly.

<u>Legal Notice:</u>

This book is copyright protected. It is only for personal use. You cannot amend, distribute, sell, use, quote or paraphrase any part, or the content within this book, without the consent of the author or publisher.

<u>Disclaimer Notice:</u>

Please note the information contained within this document is for educational and entertainment purposes only. All effort has been executed to present accurate, up to date, reliable, complete information. No warranties of any kind are declared or implied. Readers acknowledge that the author is not engaged in the rendering of legal, financial, medical or professional advice. The content within this book has been derived from various sources. Please consult a licensed professional before attempting any techniques outlined in this book.

By reading this document, the reader agrees that under no circumstances is the author responsible for any losses, direct or indirect, that are incurred as a result of the use of the information contained within this document, including, but not limited to, errors, omissions, or inaccuracies.

TABLE OF CONTENTS

Introduction

Who is ready to feel better, lose weight and improve your overall health in a sustainable way? I imagine quite a few hands raised on that question, because we all have some kind of goal in mind when it comes to our bodies, but we're uncertain how to get there. You may hear different fads or trends being tossed around and are skeptical of how well they work, so you continue in your bad habits, leery of every new ideology that comes about. This book can equip you with the information on one of those common trends today so that you can make a better evaluation as to whether this is something you should pursue.

Have you ever heard of the keto diet? In our modern culture, it has gained popularity. Many people swear by it. When you ask someone what it's all about, they might give you a list of cheats or talk about the foods that they can still eat. That is fine, but it does not do much to define what the diet actually is. Someone talking about foods they can have is not really helpful to a person who cannot have those foods. It's more helpful to explain the framework of the diet to give people more control over how this might work in their own life. This allows them to take the principles and apply them in a way that is individualized to that particular person's needs, goals, or preferences.

This book is designed to give a basic overview of the ketogenic diet so that you can have a working understanding of what that truly means and make a decision on what is right for you. A well-informed decision is a good decision. We are not going to focus on all the ways to cheat the system or get around the diet, because we feel that would not help you achieve your goals. If that is what you are looking for, this may not be the book for you. Our goal is to prepare you with the foundational knowledge of the ketogenic diet to make your own decisions without trying to force you in a particular direction or teach you ways to cut corners. A lot of resources on the ketogenic diet today promote ways to "cheat" the diet so you learn more about the loopholes than you do about what actually is supposed to make this diet work. You need to have a strong foundational understanding of how something works before trying to work around the system. Hopefully this book will help you create that foundation so that you are able to connect the commonly used terms to their definitions to decipher how the diet actually works. People tend to not try diets that they do not believe will work. Our goal is not to sway you to partake in this diet if you truly feel that it is not right for you, but to show the mechanics and science of how the diet goes into action.

We all want to be our best, healthiest selves, but we are also busy people. We want to know whether a project or activity is worth our time. This book will help you evaluate the keto diet for yourself and come to your own conclusion.

Chapter 1: So What Is the Keto Diet Anyway?

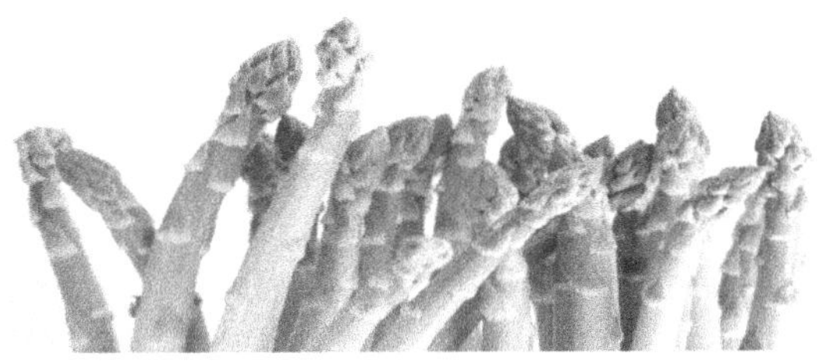

It seems like the keto diet has almost become a new buzz word in the health and fitness industry. A lot of people have promoted the diet, and many restaurants are even jumping on the bandwagon, selling items that are keto friendly to accommodate health-conscious patrons. This may have sparked your curiosity as to what this diet actually entails. Is it as healthy as people claim? Does it really work as well as people enthusiastically declare? The ketogenic diet or the keto diet is a plan that limits carbs and promotes a higher proportion of healthy fats. According to experts, the reduction in the carb intake is what propels the body into an accelerated fat-burning state. That accelerated state of fat burning is the goal you want to reach, because that is where the majority of the benefits occur. This state is referred to as *ketosis*. There are different versions of this low-carb, high-fat diet. You have the standard ketogenic diet, cyclical ketogenic diet, targeted ketogenic diet, and high protein ketogenic diet. They all have the same general concept of the low-carb and high-fat, but with slight variations. The standard ketogenic diet "is very low carb, moderate protein, and high fat" (Mawer, 2020). The cyclical ketogenic diet includes periods of refueling with more carbs, "such as 5 ketogenic days followed by 2 high carb days" (Mawer,2020). The targeted ketogenic diet gives you the freedom to incorporate more carbs around the time of your workouts to replenish the body. The high protein ketogenic diet is comparable to the standard that most people will partake in, but they add in additional portions of protein. "The ratio is often 60% fat, 35% protein, and 5% carbs" (Mawer, 2020). In each version, you can see how the fat portion is always the largest part of the diet. It should be noted that the cyclical and targeted versions are typically ones that you would find an invested athlete partaking in, participating in rigorous training such as bodybuilding, weightlifting, and HIIT.

Ketosis

We have all probably heard someone at this point rave about their results while on the keto diet. The ideology of the ketogenic diet revolves around getting your body into this heightened fat burning state known as ketosis. Once there, you will begin reaping the benefits. To get into ketosis, you are switching your body's common fuel sources in order to make your metabolism operate differently. Once your body makes the switch, it will turn your body into an efficient fat-burning machine, but the key is to maintain this state. This will generally occur when you drastically limit your intake of carbs, causing your body to have to rely on fats and ketones for sustenance. You are technically in ketosis when your blood possesses a high percentage of ketones.

Ketones are tiny molecules of fuel that your body produces that people rely on for energy when on this diet. "When you eat very few carbs or very few calories, your body produces ketones from fat" (Eenfeldt, 2021). The keto diet is not the only way to reach ketosis, but is the most effective way. People who are diabetic will sometimes reach ketosis because their blood sugar levels are low. While the desire is to keep glucose levels low for ketosis, it can be dangerous if blood sugar falls too low, and ketones in the blood becomes too high, which is known as diabetic ketoacidosis. The reason you are cutting back on the carb intake is to reduce the glucose that your body consumes. When your body is consuming glucose, it will use that for fuel rather than burning fat, meaning your body will not reduce the fat as quickly as you would like. The body can synthesize glucose from protein as well, which is why those levels need to be monitored as well.

Ketosis allows your body to transition its energy source in a way that is more sustainable without energy spikes or pitfalls. To stay in ketosis, you have to be mindful of the ingredients that are in the food you are eating. To determine whether you have actually reached the state of ketosis, there are some symptoms that you can look for, including higher frequency of urination, unquenchable thirst, and reduced appetite. Something to keep in mind is that ketosis may be more of a challenge to reach depending on your body type, your medical history, and your self-discipline.

People can also get into ketosis by intermittent fasting. Intermittent fasting is when you limit your eating to a narrow time frame. When you are not in that window, you abstain from eating. A common way of fasting is by doing the 16:8, which is 16 hours of fasting and an eight hour eating window. There are also alternate day fasts, meaning you eat only on certain days. The whole premise is that you would eat all your meals within that allotted eating window. This helps people get into ketosis because the fasting period allows the body to properly digest food and then revert to stored fat for energy. Individuals have found decent results by coupling the keto diet with intermittent fasting to better support their weight loss and health goals that they have.

Fuel Sources

What sets the keto diet apart from other diets is its effectiveness to bring the body into ketosis and keep it there. In a typical diet, the body relies on carbs as its main fuel source. These are then broken down into glucose, which is sugar that becomes usable to the body. To maintain ketosis, you have to take away or severely minimize the glucose supply to force your body to supply its energy from fat, whether that is from stored fat off of your body or fat that is eaten through your diet.

Depending on which version of the ketogenic diet you follow, you will need to monitor your daily intake of fats, protein and carbs. The fat intake needs to be the largest percentage consumed each day, and to promote a healthy lifestyle, you will want to have those fats be on the healthier side such as monounsaturated fats. We will talk more in depth about healthy fats versus toxic fats in the next chapter. Since you are wanting to lower your glucose level, you will also need to eliminate most sugars, since they will move you out of ketosis. It's a challenge, because sugar hides in so many foods, not just desserts. It is up to the dieter to read through ingredient lists and eliminate any foods that contain sugar.

The major fuel sources for your body on the keto diet are ketones and glycogen. These are your body's way of compensating to use its own storage for fuel instead of relying on food. When people eat a high-carb diet, it allows the body to become more complacent, not working to use its resources. By switching to the keto diet, this makes your body use what it has been given and increase its productivity in fat-burning.

Your brain requires a lot of energy to function. It typically uses glucose, but when that is not available, it will use the ketones from your body fat to propel it forward. Another source that is used is glycogen. Glycogen is stored in the body after eating carbohydrates that are converted to glucose. Any leftover glucose is "linked together in chains of eight to twelve glucose units which form a glycogen molecule" (Dolson, 2006). Glycogen stored in the muscles will be used for those particular areas of the body, while organs like the liver have stores of glycogen the entire body can tap into.

Chapter 2: How to Sustain the Keto Diet

The ketogenic diet requires you to be on top of your food intake, making sure that each meal is apportioned appropriately. Many people start this diet with the best of intentions. They are excited to reap the benefits but do not consider how this will look long-term, which is not uncommon in the health and fitness industry. While some dietary trends can allow you to see results quickly and keep those results with minimal changes to your daily life, the ketogenic diet does not work quite the same way. The general goal of the keto diet is ketosis, and it takes some diligence before you can reach that point where you can start cashing in on these rewards that everyone gushes over. When you get out of ketosis, you cannot just hop back in whenever you feel like it. There is a process that you have to go through to prepare your body by diligently fueling your body correctly until your body starts using its own stores for energy. If you eat low-carb some days and whatever you like on other days, you won't reach ketosis. Depending on the time span of eating and what was eaten, you might never reach ketosis, which means you are putting yourself through this cycle without seeing any progress. At this point, you may get frustrated and think that the diet is not for you because it is not working, when the truth is you just need to push a little farther to reach ketosis. To see the progress and health benefits, sustaining the diet is key.

You need to know when you are in ketosis. You can be observant of the symptoms that you are showcasing and cross reference against the lists of symptoms of individuals in ketosis. Since some of the symptoms can be general and could be indicative of other ailments, you want to consider taking a test to double check. There are tests that are available at either your local drugstore or at some grocery stores.

Depending on your comfort level, you have three main options for the tests: urine, breath or blood tests. These tests detect the presence of ketones in your body. You have to reach a certain level of ketones before you are technically considered in ketosis. While we have been talking primarily about ketones being present in the blood, the truth of the matter is that if you are in ketosis, there will be no hiding it. You will exhibit ketones in many areas of your body, which is why multiple tests can still give you an accurate reading. You are not able to compare each test to each other because each one is designed to find a specific ketone in that area of your body.

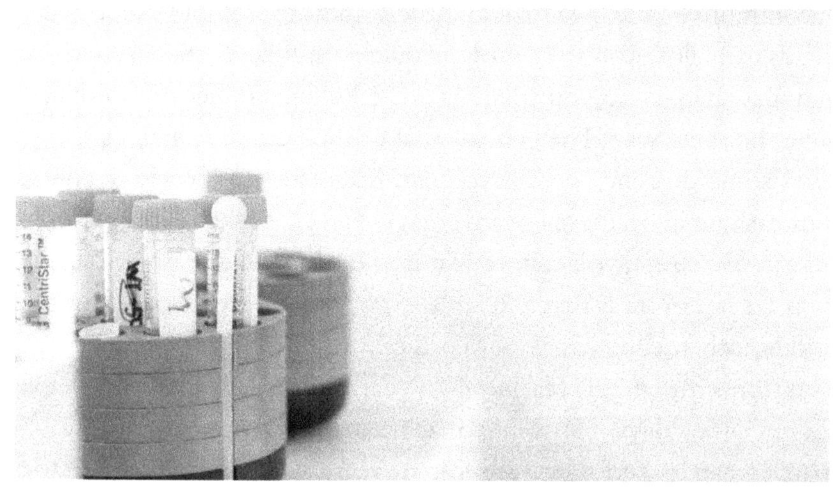

If you choose the blood ketone meter, you will have to prick your finger to extract the blood. If you use the breath meter, there are many different models and versions available, so you will need to hunt through the options to find what is best for you. Once you have the breath meter you want, you will be given instructions to use your diaphragm muscles to push every ounce of air out of your lungs for assessment. Urine tests are similar to pregnancy tests in that you are given a strip that you will need to urinate on or dip into urine in order to get a reading of what is present in your body. Most of the urine tests are similar in design and are among the easier, less invasive options for testing.

You must know how to fuel your body. That is the case for any diet you want to take part in. Before we go into the specifics of different foods and culinary options, we are going to break down the food categories that have been mentioned earlier which are protein, fats, and carbs. Why are these so important? How do they affect your diet?

Types of Macros

You will hear this term quite a bit when on this diet. Macros or macronutrients are not to be confused with micronutrients. "Macronutrients are big picture nutrition categories, such as carbohydrates, fats, and proteins. Micronutrients are smaller nutritional categories, such as individual vitamins and minerals like calcium, zinc, and vitamin B-6" (Nall, 2019). The ketogenic is focused on measuring the macros that you intake daily. This is not to diminish the value of the micronutrients, but entering into ketosis is dependent on how you structure your consumption of carbohydrates, fats and proteins. Fats are an excellent source of energy, particularly in times when food or sustenance is scarce. Dietary fat is a necessary part of your overall health. "Fat is "necessary for insulation, proper cell function, and protection of vital organs" (Dolson, 2006). In decades past, fat received a bad reputation as food companies were promoting fat free products and the idea is that these are healthier for you than the original versions. When the fat is completely taken out of a product, it is usually replaced with synthetic ingredients that offer very little in terms of nutrition and can even be worse than the fat it is replacing. Because of this ideology that was so heavy in diet culture, there is still a stigma against eating fat, but contrary to popular belief, fats are very good for you as long as you are consuming the right kinds.

Protein is essential for muscle development, and we use our muscles for all of our daily functions. How the protein benefits the muscles is that it feeds the body amino acids that are then used for the formation of muscles and to support major organs. While your body can create several amino acids on its own, it cannot create all of them, so it's up to you to make up the deficit through your diet and keep your body healthy. Those amino acids that are reliant on your food are more commonly referred to as the *essential* amino acids. There are different types of proteins: incomplete and complete. This refers to the types of amino acids that are present in that specific protein.

Carbohydrates, or carbs for short, are the major energy source for your body. When your body needs fuel, its default is to burn carbs that have been eaten that day. Your body does this naturally because it's less work to make the necessary conversions. It is only after these stores are not available that it will switch to ketones and fat for sustenance.

There are two basic types of carbs: complex and simple. Simple carbs are designed to be used quickly by the body for immediate energy. These will give a quick boost that will be diminished in the short term. Complex carbs are built more intricately "long strings of sugar units that take longer for the body to break down and use" (Dolson, 2021). Instead of being used immediately, complex carbs siphon out energy over a longer duration of time. Complex carbs provide a more even distribution of fuel that does not cause large drops in energy that are commonly seen with simple carbs. They also have a positive effect on digestion and maintaining healthy cholesterol.

Why There is No "Essential Carbohydrate"

Carbohydrates are a large part of most diets, especially in American culture. You will not see a no-carb diet, and if you do, it will not be one that can be sustained for the long term. There is no denying that carbs are a well-loved food group. All carbs that are consumed are used to fuel your body. Your body will generally use carbs for energy for its accessibility, but carbs are not required in order to fuel the body.

Some reluctance people have with any low carb diet is they believe reducing carbs is not healthy, which is contrary to evidence. Many studies and countless testimonials show that low-carb diets benefit health. The fact that this type of diet can be sustained further verifies that you can maintain a healthy lifestyle without an inordinate amount of carbs. With protein, there are amino acids that are essential, but there are no essential carbohydrates. That is because carbohydrates are not necessary for survival. The human body will revert to backup sources of energy and will find ways to replenish itself if the carb intake is low. That is one of the wonders of the human body. It is resilient enough to make up for any lack of supplies or nutrition. A majority of meals encompass a huge quantity of carbs, but that tends to be more from preference and convenience. Comfort foods that people enjoy typically have a lot of carbs. In our busy lives, people are looking for quick solutions to their hunger, so fast food restaurants and food delivery services have been frequented where there are not a lot of healthy options being offered. The USDA food pyramid, which many students were taught in American schools, was designed to teach us how to portion our food groups. The largest section at the bottom of the pyramid was the bread, cereal, rice, and pasta group, indicating that carbs should be the food group that you consume the largest amount of each day. From an early age, we are instructed to think that if we do not have a high intake of carbs over all the other food groups, we will not be healthy. That is a false claim, and it is important to dismantle this belief so you are able to fully grasp the effectiveness of a low-carb diet.

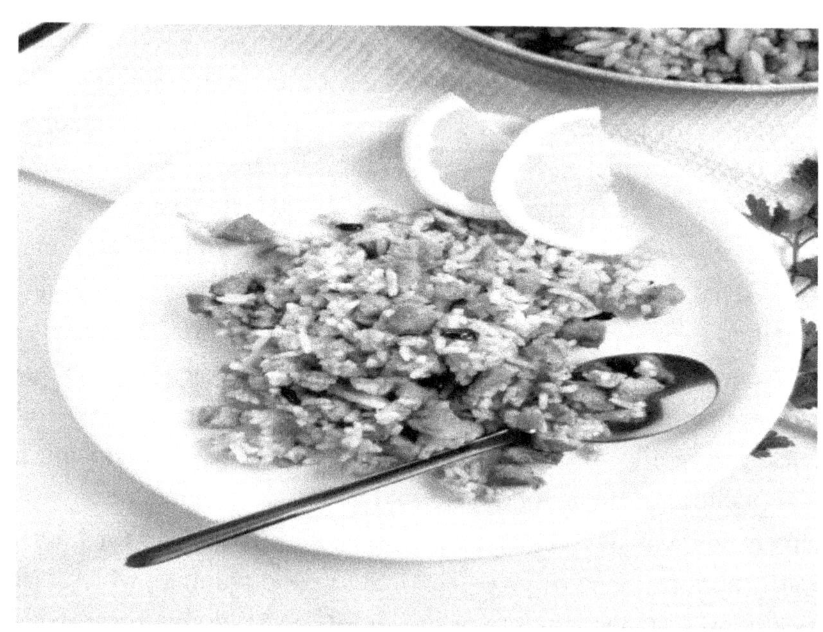

Healthy Fats Vs. Toxic Fats

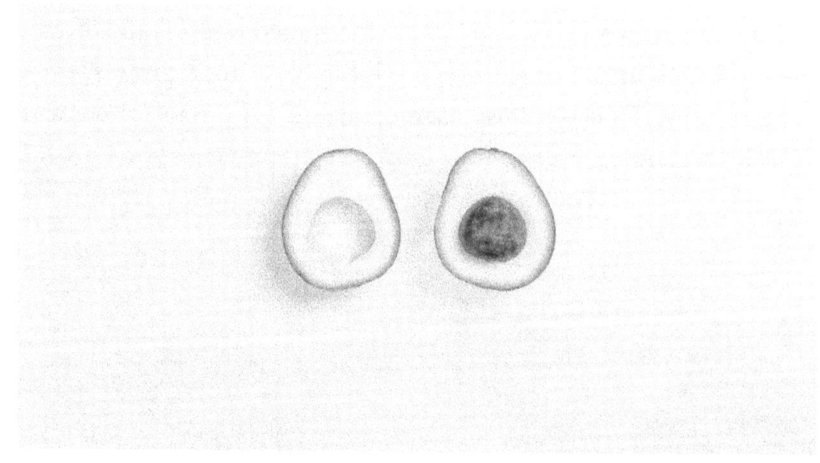

The keto diet is a high fat and low carb plan, but before you start stuffing your face with bacon, we need to recognize that not all fats are worth the same nutritional value. There are fats that are considered healthy which are monounsaturated and polyunsaturated. Then there are fats that are considered unhealthy and should be avoided if possible. Those are saturated and trans fats. Trans fats are actually the worst type of fat for your heart and can spike inflammation across the body. Inflammation is typically the underlying cause for a number of illnesses and ailments. Trans fats are found in partially hydrogenated vegetable oils often used to cook fried foods and baked goods. Saturated fats can raise cholesterol levels to an unsafe level, which can create a slippery slope of other medical problems. They are found in fatty animal proteins and full fat-dairy foods. Consuming unhealthy fats on a regular basis is detrimental for your health and encapsulates what people envision when they desire to eliminate fat from their diet. However, to completely get rid of all fat from your diet would also rob you of the benefits that healthy fats have to offer. Both monounsaturated and polyunsaturated fats improve cholesterol levels while decreasing the risk of heart disease.

CHAPTER 3: BENEFITS OF A KETOGENIC DIET

Anyone who starts a diet is hoping to improve their body and health. A good way to evaluate a new lifestyle change is by looking over the pros and cons. When deciding on which diet is best for you, you may be inclined to want to know what the benefits are to help you determine. These can then be compiled onto the pros side for each idea so after you are done, you can look at each plan objectively.

The ketogenic diet boasts a wide range of benefits. That is what draws people to the diet in the first place, and the benefits tend to be what motivates people to continue pursuing that change. People notice positive changes in different areas of their body that improve their quality of life. If you continue on the diet long enough, you will notice changes internally as well as externally. The diet is set up for you to see change, and if you do not, that should be cause for concern. People will gush over the dramatic physical effects that they will see. They will compare how their body functions before the diet to how it functions when they are partaking in the diet, being pleased with the improvement. There may even be areas of their body that they thought were operating just fine that will increase their productivity. Sometimes we get so accustomed to how our body has been working on the daily that we do not realize that there is still room to grow.

Anti-Inflammatory Benefits

The source of many ailments within the body is inflammation. Inflammation is part of your body's natural defense against disease, viruses, and bacteria. While its purpose is designed for good and is necessary to combat infection, chronic inflammation makes it harder for your body to function normally. You are on heightened alert, becoming more tense. Normal functions become increasingly more difficult, especially if the problem is not dealt with. If inflammation spreads to multiple parts of the body, chronic pain hinders the body from doing daily activities or anything that would help alleviate the symptoms. Inflammation is trying to push out the foreign bacteria that is present in the body and filters out the viruses that have potentially invaded. It serves as an alert that something is not right within the body, and it needs to be addressed. If the issue is ignored, it can sometimes escalate to a bigger problem. At that point, the body becomes so inflamed that it cannot effectively ward off any new ailments, so it actually becomes more susceptible to all kinds of new illnesses, diseases, and even injuries. Common symptoms include swelling, a change in color to appear more red, and pain of varying degrees.

You need to have a way to regulate the inflammation that may be present and give it an outlet in order to keep balance. The ketogenic diet helps with regulating the body systems for a couple reasons. The first reason is related to the foods you eat and don't eat. Many keto foods naturally reduce inflammation, such as cauliflower, avocados, fatty fish, eggs, and spinach. And many foods that cause inflammation, such as processed grains, sugars, starchy vegetables, and fruits that have a high level of fructose, are not part of the keto diet.

Another way that the ketogenic diet helps the body fight inflammation is it sets up the body to produce its own anti-inflammatory fighters. Ketones bolster your body's natural defenses. "What that means is that your body is producing the ketone BHB (beta-hydroxybutyrate), which has proven to be associated with activating genes that improve mitochondrial function and decrease oxidative stress. Ketosis also activates the AMPK pathway (activated protein kinase), which assists in regulating energy and inhibiting the inflammatory Nf-kB pathways" (Winters, 2021). In other words, the keto diet helps your body be more resilient against the invaders that may come into your system to compromise your health. Your body is building up its own little army to fight on your behalf to put it in simple terms.

Cognitive Benefits

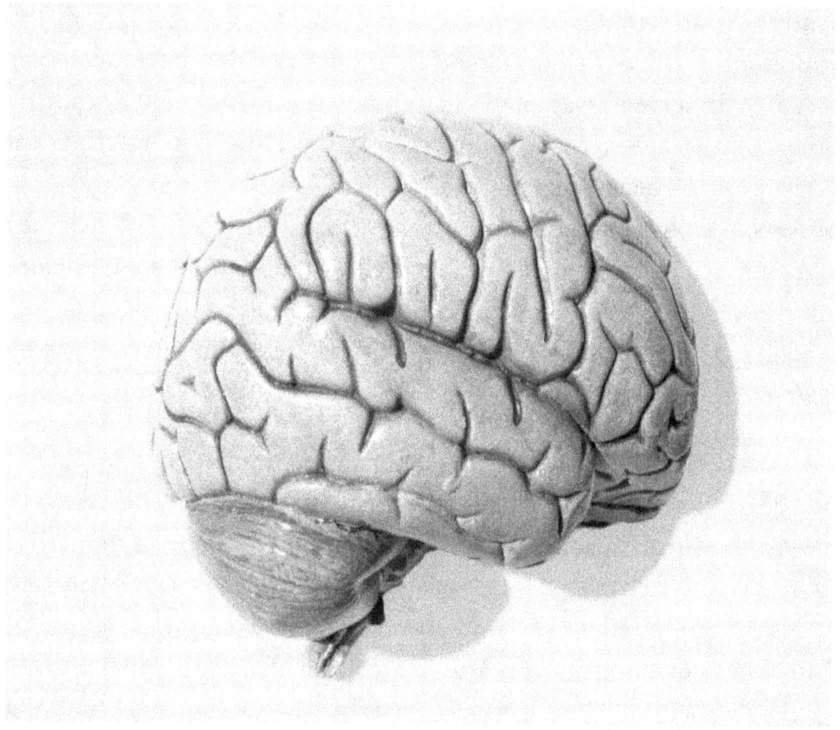

The keto diet has also been touted to provide positive changes to the brain and its performance. Those who follow the plan for an extended period notice improvement in their brain's capacity to function, making it more effective for daily tasks and ready to navigate any unexpected stressors. There are a few reasons for this diet's effectiveness, and they generally have to do with its design.

We have talked earlier in the book about the structure of the keto diet. This lowers carb intake and increases the fat intake. By supplementing the absence of additional carbs with more fat, the brain flourishes as there is improvement in brain activity. The ketones that serve as a sustainable generator of energy prove to be helpful to those whose bodies are already struggling to perform properly with glucose. Studies have noted particular improvements in individuals with Type 2 diabetes or Alzheimer's. Older individuals noticed that the symptoms of minor cognitive impairment lessened. "The production of ketone bodies can help in these cases because the brains of people with these problems can't use enough of the available glucose to handle cognition and perception" (Godinez, 2016). The supplementation of ketones takes some strain off of a body that is already having difficulty functioning normally, providing the brain energy to perform better. There is some belief that the keto diet is an excellent way to cope with epilepsy as well. Epilepsy is basically erratic brain activity where the brain has trouble processing information, resulting in seizures. Some people will only have the illness for a season of their life, while others experience seizures for the majority of their lives . Currently there is no cure, so sufferers must manage it in their daily lives, understanding the potential for a seizure at any time. "A study completed in 2012 found that children with epilepsy following a ketogenic diet had improved alertness and cognitive functioning when compared to traditional anti-epileptic pharmacotherapeutics" (Biljon, 2019). By helping the brain function properly, keto reduces the risk of epileptic seizures to occur. Dealing with epilepsy is stressful for patients, as you often do not know when to expect them because you are given little to no warning. This can put family members on edge, and the epileptic individual often has to give up some freedoms such as driving. The keto diet brings back more of a sense of control and peace to those who are tense with worry over this condition.

The keto diet, when done well, showcases the benefit of healthy fats in the body. If you are following the protocol correctly, you will be consuming foods that are rich in the nutritious fats and essential fatty acids such as omega-3 and omega-6. These fatty acids provide much-needed nourishment to our bodies and are often lacking in our standard American diet, but if you incorporate a variety of the acceptable keto foods into your diet, you can build your consumption of these vital nutrients. Along with supporting the body, omega-3 and omega-6 provide specific nutrients to help your brain improve its function because they are crucial building blocks to brain development.

People on the keto diet notice improved mental clarity. Ever have those days when you are struggling to think clearly, or your brain is sluggish to think of responses in the middle of a conversation? This is brain fog, and we have all experienced it at some point. Tasks we could normally do without batting an eye now require more focus. Having to concentrate more on the simplest tasks leaves you with less energy to handle larger, more complex activities. Brain fog can occur for a number of reasons, such as fatigue, stress, inadequate sleep, or improper diet. The reason that the diet can be a cause is that the brain is not getting the necessary nutrients it needs to perform its required tasks, so it is essentially starving of its essential vitamins, minerals and nutritional support. Imagine yourself when you are hungry and have not eaten in several hours or maybe even days. Your stomach is rumbling, your motivation level is low, your strength is not where it normally is, and you have less control over your faculties such as emotions. The same is true with our brains when they are hungry for nutrients. A neurotransmitter called glutamate is crucial for how your brain operates. Brain fog occurs if there is too much glutamate present in the brain, so when you are on the keto diet and in ketosis, the ketones give the body some backup to filter through the excess glutamate so that you can continue functioning relatively normally. On top of improving mental clarity, memory is sharper as well.

Other Health Benefits

Along with cognitive and anti-inflammatory benefits, there are other positives to be considered by this diet as well. If you are looking to improve your health, this might be a plan to consider because of the list of benefits that it can produce. An area that this diet improves upon is body fat percentage. This diet helps people to burn through their fat storage more effectively because they are utilizing their own body makeup to provide them with energy rather than defaulting to the glucose created by the food ingested. Lower body fat reduces joint pain and improves mobility because it lessens the stress placed on the joints from having to carry a larger load. This allows a person to be more active, and exercise is part of a healthy lifestyle to mitigate the chance of disease. Lower body fat reduces the chance of diseases such as Type 2 diabetes and heart disease because increased body fat is a contributing factor in these ailments. When body fat is reduced, the body does not have to work as hard to pump blood to every area. High body fat is hazardous to your health in general, so eliminating that risk factor alone has a positive impact on your well-being.

The keto diet also improves or eliminates symptoms of multiple illnesses and ailments, including Parkinson's disease and polycystic ovary syndrome (PCOS). With PCOS, research suggests the keto diet helps balance hormones. Individuals have remarked on lessened effects of their Parkinson's symptoms, making the disease more tolerable in their daily life. There is still work being done to determine keto's effects on cancer, but the research that has been collected seems to be favorable in decreasing the speed at which cancer spreads throughout the body. The keto diet appears to help individuals ease back into normalcy after suffering from different brain injuries by reducing the long-term impact. There is still more research to be done in order for these results to be conclusive.

Chapter 4: MythBusters

We have now heard the positives of the ketogenic diet which are hard to ignore, but now we must address the rumors around this fad. There is so much information being thrown out these days that it can be hard to filter through it all. You want to make an informed decision, and the benefits of keto sure make it tempting, but there are those pesky myths looming in your mind that we should address to give you a wider picture. We do not want you to base your decision off of fear. The best way to help you is to arm you with information that tackles these common beliefs about the keto diet.

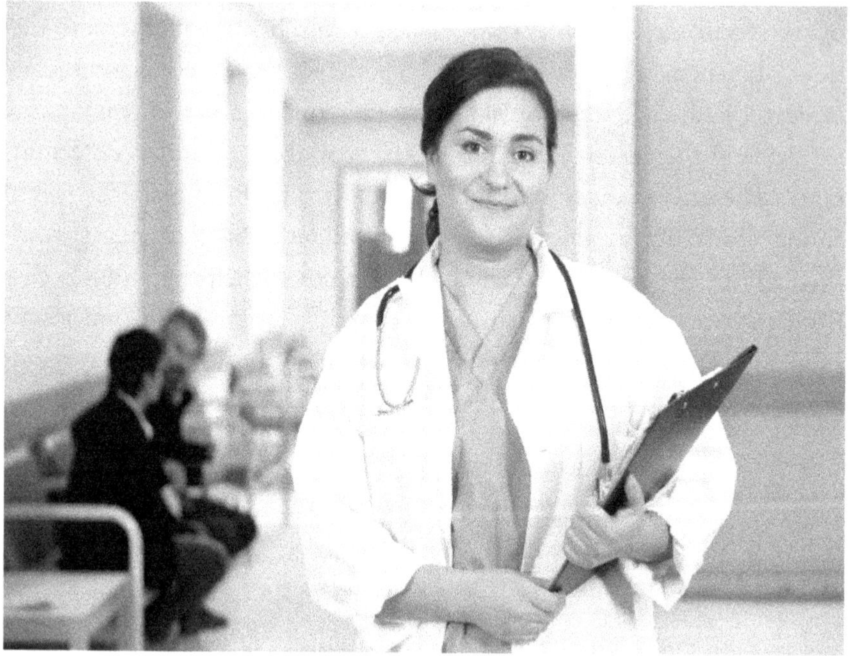

The first myth we will address is ketosis and ketoacidosis are interchangeable. That is not true. Ketosis deals with how your body is fueling itself. It switches from being reliant on glucose to ketones and fat so that your body is burning through your fat for fuel. This is where you want to be if you are in the keto diet, and it is not harmful. This is not to be confused with ketoacidosis. "Ketoacidosis is a potentially life-threatening state in which the body's blood is highly acidic and is most often seen with people with diabetes" (Yannone, 2018). If anyone is steering clear of the keto diet because they believe that they will get ketoacidosis, they are misinformed. To suggest this would be to say that the diet would cause harm to the blood, and there is far too much research on the benefits of keto to suggest that the blood would reach a dangerous level.

The second myth is that you are free to eat whatever type of fat that you like. There are two ways to approach this myth. While you are increasing the fat intake for your proportions, simply being on a diet does not absolve you from the consequences of making the food choices that you do. The foods still contain the same nutritional value regardless of whether you eat them on their own or part of a diet. If they are low in nutrition, they will most likely not help you toward your goals. Doctors will advise individuals who are deciding to partake in the keto diet to focus on healthy fats and drastically reduce or cut intake of saturated fats. However, there are people who will partake in the keto diet with what is called a dirty keto where they are a bit looser with the restrictions and will often allow themselves to eat any kind of fat. They still maintain the basic principles of the proportions in order to get the physical results they are wanting, but they may not have as many benefits as someone who is diligently following every protocol. Medical professionals will advise against high consumption of saturated fats because this is detrimental to a person's overall health and most likely negate the reasons a person partakes in the diet in the first place. Technically, you can still do the keto diet by consuming any kind of fat. However, proponents of keto don't recommend it.

The next myth is that your brain can operate at its absolute best without the consumption of carbs. To get to the cognitive benefits of the keto diet, it will require some perseverance to get there. Those goals will not be reached overnight. Your body will also need time to adapt to the change, especially if your lifestyle prior to keto was drastically different than what you are doing now. While your body transitions from burning carbs to burning fat, your brain will not be operating optimally. "In the process of becoming fat adapted, people may experience the same symptoms they do when they are "hangry" or passing the time before their lunch break. Once the body becomes fat adapted the brain can convert ketones as fuel, but White says that this can take weeks to months to finally happen" (Yannone, 2018). Do not walk into this diet expecting to see immediate changes. In the beginning, you can expect to feel a bit sluggish, irritable, slower in reflexes, and possibly have a lowered motivation to participate in things. This is not to say that the keto diet does not help your brain function, because doctors have seen a correlation between the diet and improved brain activity.

Another myth is that you can seesaw on your diet and still manage to hold off the weight. In general, going back and forth with your weight is not great for your body. It creates extra stress on your body as it adjusts to more weight and then quickly removing it. Yo-yoing on your diet can hinder your metabolism. Metabolism is the way that your body takes the food and drink you consume to then transform into usable energy. Having a healthy metabolism means that your body is utilizing the calories efficiently to the point where there is not a large excess. There is a cycle and your body is functioning properly. If your metabolism is not working well, that means that your body takes very few calories from food for energy. This makes it harder for a person to burn fat and calories because the body is slower at processing them than the person is at consuming them, allowing the calories to build up to the point where the body cannot burn off the excess.

With the keto diet, you have to work to get into ketosis so that you can get into the fat burning mode. This takes time. You are telling your brain and body to change its default for energy. Imagine taking the time to set that up, getting into ketosis, seeing results, dropping the diet for a short time, and then trying to pick it back up immediately.

You then have to start over to get back into ketosis. It becomes a pattern as someone will enter into the fat burning state, stopping and starting all over again. This can be confusing for your body to figure out where to get its energy, so it could be taking it longer to burn fat and lose weight each new time you restart keto. If you seesaw on the diet, you cannot expect to keep the results consistently because you are not even being consistent with your process. It takes time and hard work to lose weight. It takes similar effort to maintain that weight loss.

The next myth we will address is that the keto diet is the best way out there to lose weight today. We need to understand that everybody is different, which sounds a bit like a cliché, but we each have a unique genetic makeup. Our bodies are each designed with their own specific types of metabolism, allergies, and preferences. What works for one group of people may prove to be ineffective for another group. If we say that this is the best way to lose weight, then people will desperately focus only on this plan, when in reality, there are a myriad of resources and options to lose weight.

Some people may find that what works best for them is a hybrid of a few plans or diets. Part of what works with the keto diet is going into ketosis. There are other ways to reach ketosis such as intermittent fasting. There is no one way better than others to lose weight because weight loss is nuanced. It depends on a number of factors such as age, activity level, health and hormones. If two people doing the exact same diet do not have the same results, it goes back to their individual bodily makeup. Pre-existing conditions or diseases within a person's body can also affect their ability to lose weight.

Claiming that keto is the best diet for weight loss can also promote a problem by setting expectations too high, so then people will start the plan with lofty goals, and when they aren't met quickly, they will throw in the towel before their body has really had time to adapt to the changes. If they did not lose weight with this plan, they are less motivated to try others. If keto is supposedly the best diet, and it didn't work, what hope is there for other diets that are not as popular?

When we look at someone's weight loss on keto, we should also take into consideration what their activity level was like, because that will affect the amount of calories that were burned to create the desired weight loss. People can make dramatic changes to their appearance with diet alone, but do not be surprised if many have coupled some kind of exercise regimen with their diet to bolster the effects.

Chapter 5: How to Begin

Before you start the keto diet, you will need to make some preparations and make sure that you are set up for success. If you just jump into the diet without a plan, you will not last long because you will not have the necessary materials or know what to do when something unexpected arises. Of course, you cannot predict all of life's surprises, but having a plan keeps you more grounded and prevents you from shifting off-course to grab something less healthy. This would be a good time to evaluate what is currently in your pantry. We will be looking over what foods to avoid, what foods are okay on the ketogenic diet, and we will even give tips on how to plan out meals. With this information, you can determine what you need to do before starting. For the best results, it is best to get rid of the non-keto foods so you are not prone to grabbing them when you get stressed or are feeling lazy. You can then replace them with foods and snacks that are acceptable in the diet and supportive of your goals.

What To Avoid

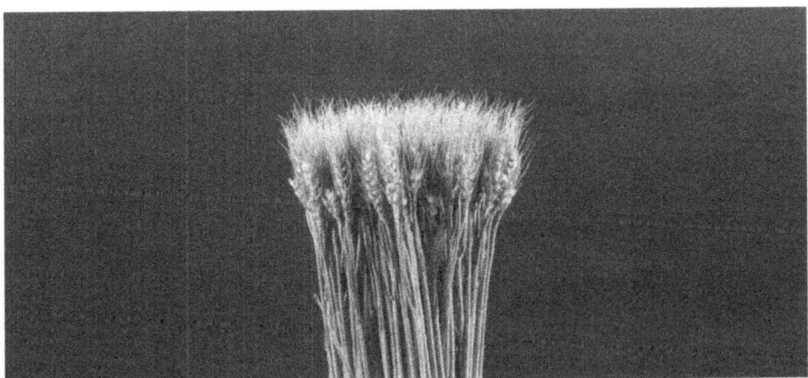

This is probably not going to be your favorite section of the book, but it is necessary. You will need to avoid grains and starches. There are several types of grains out there such as barley, amaranth, wheat, rye, and oats. Grains are the main ingredients in breads, pastas, oatmeal, crackers, cereal, and most granola. With starches, that means you are avoiding potatoes, root vegetables and legumes. Root vegetables include parsnips and carrots. Legumes will include lentils, beans, chickpeas and peas. You will also need to avoid alcohol and sugars. This may be difficult for those who enjoy having a drink or dessert as a stress reliever, so this could be a reason to find a healthier option to manage emotions and stress. Also avoid foods advertised as sugar free, because they generally are sweetened with artificial sweeteners and are highly processed. Since this is a diet that is focusing on increasing the fat intake, you want to avoid food items that are lower in fat or no fat because that will go against one of the principles of the diet. This may sound surprising, but you will need to avoid fruit as well except minimal amounts of berries from time-to-time. The reason is because of the natural sugars that are present inside many fruits.

Foods That Are Safe To Eat

To contrast what you cannot eat on this diet, let us now focus on the foods that are acceptable while being ketogenic. All meat is acceptable. To ensure better quality, you may want to look for grass fed or free range, but that is not required. This includes fatty fish, which contains healthy fats that are strongly encouraged while on keto. In general, seafood is acceptable on this diet. You are able to have dairy such as butter, cheese, and cream. In order for it to be compliant, it will need to be full-fat and not have any added sugar. You are able to have vegetables, but you will need to be selective and only consume low-carb, non-starchy vegetables. Some examples of vegetables that are keto approved are spinach, tomatoes, cauliflower, broccoli, peppers and anything leafy. You are welcome to and advised to add in healthy fats to your daily intake as well. You can get healthy fats from avocados, olive oil, and coconut oil as a starting place. If you are on the keto diet, you can rest assured because you are still able to keep your morning cup of coffee or tea. You just may have to make a few adjustments because you will not be able to have any sweetener except limited amounts of monk fruit sweetener, so if you are used to loading your coffee with whipped cream and syrups, you will need to learn to appreciate coffee in a simpler form.

How To Plan Meals

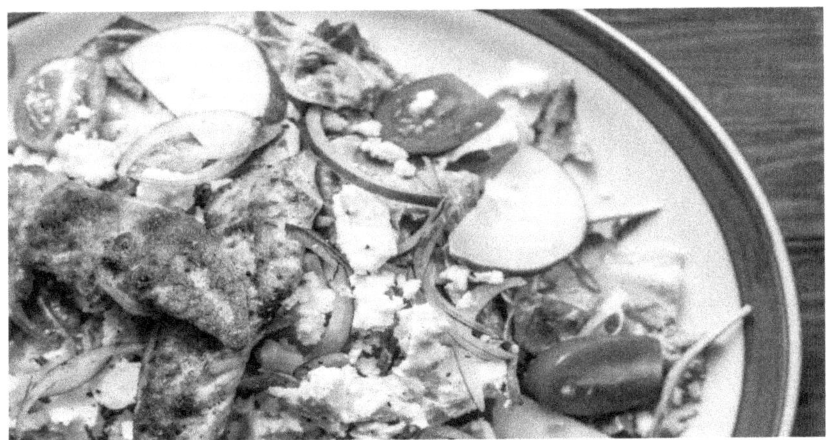

Like we mentioned earlier, having a plan is setting yourself up for success. With a diet like keto that restricts you from eating a lot of foods that you would run across on an average day, you cannot just aimlessly throw the diet together, hope for the best, and expect to see long-lasting results. What are you going to do on those days when you feel unmotivated or tired? You are not going to want to put in the effort to create a meal that is compliant and will be more likely to pick whatever the easiest, quickest option despite the fact that the option might not be the healthiest.

Write out a menu for the week. Some people will do this in a blank journal. You could also include this in your daily planner if you have one or print off sheets of a blank calendar. For each day, write out the meal you are intending to eat for breakfast, lunch and dinner. If you need ideas on keto meals, Pinterest is a good place to start for ideas or a simple Google search. It should be noted as well that it is okay to have a meal more than once. For example, if you anticipate lots of leftovers with one of your meals, you can have the leftovers the next day. Just make sure to indicate that on the menu. Having leftovers will free up time in case you are unable to cook those days as well. Once you have this plan, you can create your grocery list and stock a few keto approved snacks as well. This helps you stay on course so that you are going into the store with a specific mission and are less likely to buy items that will not contribute to your goals. Once you have purchased your items, meal prepping is your friend. Find a day to make a lot of items of the week in bulk, so that way the foods you are supposed to be eating are more easily accessible during a busy week.

Chapter 6: What To Expect When Starting The Ketogenic Diet

Everyone loves dreaming about their perfect body or their perfect health, especially when they partake in a new diet. It makes them long for that day when that dream becomes a reality. However, being fixated on that end goal can cause some people to feel blindsided when things do not happen in the timeline they expect or changes occur that they did not anticipate. The ketogenic diet can offer wonderful results for those who choose to follow the regimen properly, but like with any change, your body needs time to adjust, and you cannot expect results overnight. This diet in particular requires special diligence to keep yourself in ketosis because that is where the majority of the sought after benefits start taking place, so we should not lose heart when the progress we were so desperately hoping for is taking a bit longer to appear. As long as you persevere and continue to follow the protocol faithfully, you will see results.

Physical Changes

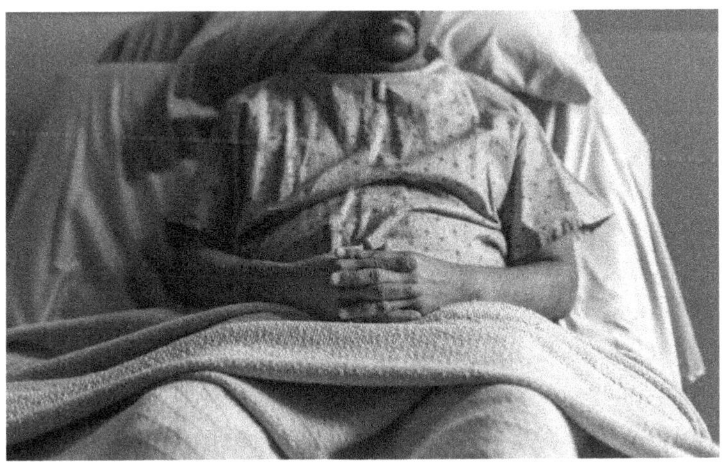

You should expect to see some physical changes with this diet. You might suffer from something called the "keto flu." This generally takes place in people who are doing their first experience with low carb or no carb diets. It is part of the body's way of adjusting to the new lifestyle with restricted carbs. Sufferers will note having symptoms that mirror the regular flu such as nausea, muscle cramps, weakness, headaches, and diarrhea. The body is under stress and will need time to resume functioning normally. Keto flu does not happen to everyone, and typically does not last long. Most people who endure this indicate that they have only had the symptoms last a week, but some individuals have commented on the symptoms lingering for a longer period of time. To combat the keto flu, it is recommended to maintain hydration, replenish lost electrolytes, keep exercise light, and make sure that you are getting enough sleep. You will also need to monitor your proportions to make sure that fat and carb intake are where they should be for the diet to be as consistent as you can to help your body adjust more quickly.

Another physical change is reduction of body fat. Since the diet is burning through fat on the body, you will start to notice the amount decreasing over the body. However the areas that you will most likely first notice the change is the midsection, thighs and any other part of the body that has a large quantity of body fat. The body will work to use that fat, as that will give it a larger store to work through. Over time, you will notice a change throughout the whole body, but it will be a gradual process.

Your body is also slimming down due to water weight loss. People typically document losing several pounds relatively soon after starting the keto diet which is incredibly motivating for people to continue. Your body is in the process of transforming into a more effective machine and part of that includes letting go of any excess. Water weight in the body is also connected to the glucose molecules or carbs present. "In general, for every 1 gram of carbs you store, you'll store 3-4 grams of water to go with it" ("5 Things to Know about Water,

Hydration, and Electrolytes on Keto"). Your body is geared towards operating off carbs because that is less effort on your body, so because of this, you are naturally storing up water weight to accompany those carbs that are then turned into glucose. Anyone who is not restricting carbs will be doing this. Even people who are restricting carb intake but not doing so correctly can accumulate more water within the body. In the first week or so, your body is not getting the amount of carbs that it is used to. With less carbs, that means there is less glucose in the body. The body will hold the water weight for a couple days to prepare for the normal carbs that it usually anticipates. When it recognizes that those carbs are not coming, the body will release the superfluous water because it does not have the need for that because sustenance is being obtained in other ways that do not require the storage of water in order to facilitate what needs to get done. The human body is accustomed to habits and when there are sudden changes, it will actively work to keep the body at its present point as long as possible. This is why the water weight is not lost immediately but after a few days. That is also why you want to set realistic, gradual goals that do not cause a major shock to the body so that it can be more sustainable instead of the body trying to work against you.

Mental Changes

We touched on cognitive benefits to the diet earlier because we want to drive home the point that keto diet has value to the body in more ways than simply physical. It has been documented that the keto diet improves symptoms of various diseases, particularly those that are neurological, but our quality of mental activity also improves. Poor mental health is becoming an epidemic across the globe and in the United States, especially after the accumulated stress of the 2020 pandemic. This has a cascading effect, as those with poor mental health will typically suffer with poor ratings in other areas as well, such as poor physical health, increased risk of disease, inadequate sleep, and poor job performance.

Those on the keto diet will notice positive changes to their mental health. Ole Hessen of Norway partook in the keto diet in 2017 and noted that "his rapid cycling bipolar disorder became much more stable and manageable" (Mullens, 2021). The diet supported his brain in functioning in a way that was conducive to a normal lifestyle. He noticed that the changes in the cycles of his bipolar disorder were not as drastic or debilitating. The diet was even returning energy back to him, which was helping him feel more motivated. He was able to develop interests and cultivate hobbies that were often hindered by effects of his disorder.

People have also remarked that the diet has helped them manage their depression, which they find less severe than before their lifestyle change. Their moods become more balanced and anticipated. They feel more comfortable as they begin to understand what to expect from themselves, better navigating mood swings in their daily lives. There were able to experience more fulfillment in their relationships which led to them having a more positive outlook on life itself. There are still studies to be done on this topic, but some are wondering if the reduction of glucose provides clarity for the brain. The ketones give the brain fuel and allow it to work in a way that promotes sharper focus than on just glucose. Your body will also strategize to use its resources more as it becomes more reliant on fat and ketones.

Another way that the keto diet may improve mental health is by reducing inflammation in the body. "Many mental health disorders are strongly linked to inflammation and oxidation, just like many physical illnesses are" (Mullens, 2021). When there is too much inflammation, it creates issues with how the body is supposed to process. The body can be slower in certain areas such as having synaptic responses in the brain occur at a lower rate. Inflammation is a stressor on the body that can lead to many serious ailments or illnesses if it is not controlled. There are situations where stress can actually restrict blood flow, so that is less oxygen and blood being circulated to the brain to function properly. By removing the inflammation, it reduces the symptoms caused by chronic cognitive disorders, sharpens mental clarity and relaxes the brain so that it can perform at its best.

Overall energy is heightened through the keto diet. This leads to higher motivation and better quality of life. When people have more energy, they are more likely to take care of tasks that need to get done, such as chores, unfinished tasks from their work, and projects around the house. They may even take an active part in supporting their own well-being by engaging in regular exercise and cooking healthy meals high in nutritional value. They are able to invest into their relationships and make stronger social connections while having the energy to keep up with them. Part of the reason for the energy increase is the foods that are consumed and omitted with this diet. The foods that are allowed are often naturally great for energy. The keto diet also eliminates any processed foods that tend to leave people feeling sluggish, lethargic, and unwilling to participate in anything. You may not even notice the effect that those foods have on you until you cut them out for a while to have a comparison. After being on the keto diet a while, people are able to get through their day with less assistance such as continual energy drink consumption throughout the day and find themselves more awake at the times of the day where they normally would have a dip in energy.

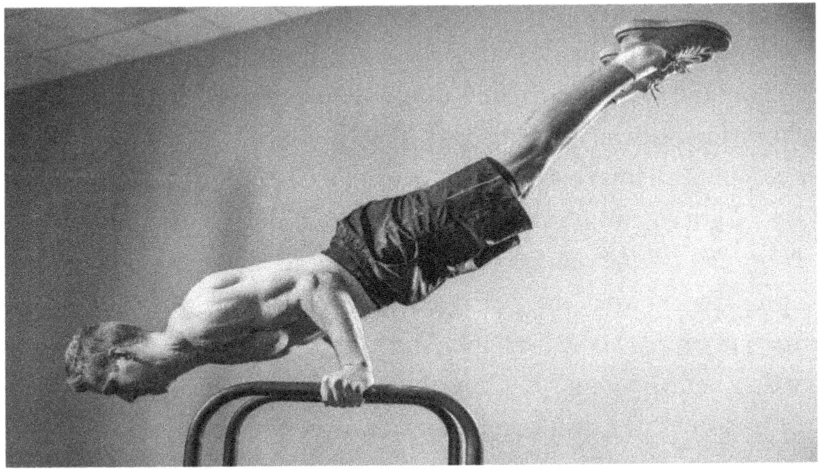

CONCLUSION

The ketogenic diet is popular because it is a different way of approaching dieting than what is out currently. While it is not new, it is regaining popularity due to extended research that allows people to better understand how to utilize the diet to serve their needs. There are several benefits to the diet that extend beyond the typical physical results that are expected of a diet. The health reasons should be cause to give this plan some attention to evaluate if this is something for you.

There are a lot of fads or weight loss items in the market today that make promises that they cannot deliver on. We see the 'get skinny' quick schemes that are destined for failure, but the keto diet is different. In principle, it is science backed to explain the methodology behind why they choose to do things a certain way. If you follow the diet carefully, you can expect to see some kind of changes. This diet promises different benefits and results that you can experience for yourself. The catch is you have to be willing to put in the work to get those results. It takes time before any of the efforts will show any fruit, but if you are able to maintain ketosis, you will reap the reward of your hard work.

If you go into the diet looking for shortcuts and loopholes to avoid living out the lifestyle correctly, don't be surprised when your outcome is far different than you expected. That is typically why people do not see results with this diet claim it does not work. This is not for the lazy. With weight loss in general, you need to put in the work. The changes will not just fall in your lap or happen without any effort on your part. Be prepared to map out a plan ahead of time. Construct a menu and write out your grocery lists, including keto-friendly snacks. If you fail to plan, then you won't last long. You will be more tempted to quit or shift to something non-compliant out of convenience. This is not to scare you away from the diet but to help you reframe your expectations to make sure that they are realistic.

If the idea is to get healthier and lose weight, you need to recognize that what you are currently doing is not getting you to those goals, which is why you probably started keto in the first place. But there is good news. Because of the popularity and increased demand for keto-friendly products, it is now easier to take on the ketogenic diet because there is a plethora of recipes, resources, and even food items at the store that are specially formulated to be compliant for the dietary plan.

We hope that this book has given you a nice overview on the keto diet. Our goal was to arm you with information to feel better about your decision to try this out or move past this diet to something else. If we have done our job well, then our goal has been met.

REFERENCES

"5 Things to Know about Water, Hydration, and Electrolytes on Keto." *Paleo Leap | Paleo Diet Recipes & Tips*, 13 Jan. 2018, paleoleap.com/5-things-need-know-water-hydration-electrolytes-keto/. Accessed 2 Apr. 2021.

Biljon, A. (2019). *The Ketogenic Diet & Brain Health*. Cognitivefxusa.com. https://www.cognitivefxusa.com/blog/the-ketogenic-diet-and-brain-health

Dolson, L. (2005, November). *Macronutrients 101*. Verywell Fit; Verywell Fit. https://www.verywellfit.com/macronutrients-2242006

Dolson, L. (2006, March 2). *The Role of Glycogen in Diet and Exercise*. Verywell Fit; Verywell Fit. https://www.verywellfit.com/what-is-glycogen-2242008

Eenfeldt, A. (2019, February 21). *Diet Doctor*. Diet Doctor. https://www.dietdoctor.com/low-carb/keto

Godinez, B. (2016, October 30). *How To Use The Ketogenic Diet for Productivity and Mental Performance*. Perfect Keto. https://perfectketo.com/use-ketogenic-diet-productivity-mental-performance/

Mawer, R. (2018). *The Ketogenic Diet: A Detailed Beginner's Guide to Keto*. Healthline. https://www.healthline.com/nutrition/ketogenic-diet-101

Mullens, A., & Ede, G. (2018, April 15). *Ketogenic diet for mental health: Come for the weight loss, stay for the mental health benefits?* Diet Doctor; Diet Doctor. https://www.dietdoctor.com/low-carb/mental-health

Nall, R. (2019, December 11). *What's the Difference Between Micronutrients and Macronutrients?* Healthline; Healthline Media. https://www.healthline.com/health/food-nutrition/micros-vs-macros

Winters, N. (2021, November 30). *How the Ketogenic Diet Reduces Inflammation.* KETO-MOJO. https://keto-mojo.com/article/keto-diet-reduces-inflammation/

Yannone, T. (2018, January 8). *5 Keto Diet Myths That You Need To Stop Believing.* Women's Health; Women's Health. https://www.womenshealthmag.com/weight-loss/a19993301/keto-diet/

PHOTOGRAPHY REFERENCES

Bradley, T. (n.d.). Wheat Grain Bundle. In *burst.shopify.com*. Retrieved April 1, 2021, from https://burst.shopify.com/photos/wheat-grain-bundle?q=grains

De Khors, N. (n.d.). Fitness Balancing. In *burst.shopify.com*. Retrieved April 1, 2021, from https://burst.shopifycdn.com/photos/fitness-balancing.jpg?width=4460&height=4460&exif=1&iptc=1

G, I. (n.d.). Fried Rice With Sliced Lemon On Ceramic Plate. In *unsplash.com*. Retrieved April 1, 2021, from https://unsplash.com/photos/UuBW0N-Lozc

Henry, M. (n.d.-a). A Man Propped Up in Hospital Bed With Hands Crossed. In *burst.shopify.com*. Retrieved April 1, 2021, from https://burst.shopifycdn.com/photos/a-man-propped-up-in-hospital-bed-with-hands-crossed.jpg?width=4460&height=4460&exif=1&iptc=1

Henry, M. (n.d.-b). Fresh Asparagus. In *burst.shopify.com*. Retrieved April 1, 2021, from https://burst.shopifycdn.com/photos/fresh-asparagus.jpg?width=4460&height=4460&exif=1&iptc=1

Henry, M. (n.d.-c). Two Avocado Slices. In *burst.shopify.com*. Retrieved April 1, 2021, from https://burst.shopifycdn.com/photos/two-avocado-slices.jpg?width=4460&height=4460&exif=1&iptc=1

Partners, S. (n.d.). A Doctor Smiles While Holding Her Clipboard. In *burst.shopify.com*. Retrieved April 1, 2021, from https://burst.shopifycdn.com/photos/a-doctor-smiles-while-

holding-her-
clipboard.jpg?width=4460&height=4460&exif=1&iptc=1

Pflug, S. (n.d.-a). Science Test Tubes. In *burst.shopify.com*. Retrieved April 1, 2021, from https://burst.shopify.com/photos/science-test-tubes?q=keto+test+strip

Pflug, S. (n.d.-b). What Does A Brain Need? In *burst.shopify.com*. Retrieved April 1, 2021, from https://burst.shopifycdn.com/photos/what-does-a-brain-need.jpg?width=4460&height=4460&exif=1&iptc=1

Vissers, B. (n.d.). Salad With Chicken. In *burst.shopify.com*. Retrieved April 1, 2021, from https://burst.shopify.com/photos/salad-with-chicken?q=dinner+plate

www.ingramcontent.com/pod-product-compliance
Lightning Source LLC
Chambersburg PA
CBHW060922130726

48001CB00006B/2361